Eating Consciously for Natural Weight Loss

By

Louistine Tuck

This book is a work of non-fiction. Names and places have been changed to protect the privacy of all individuals. The events and situations are true.

© 2003 by Louistine Tuck. All rights reserved.

No part of this book may be reproduced, stored in a retrieval system, or transmitted by any means, electronic, mechanical, photocopying, recording, or otherwise, without written permission from the author.

ISBN: 1-4107-3586-9 (e-book)
ISBN: 1-4107-3585-0 (Paperback)

Library of Congress Control Number: 2003092413

This book is printed on acid free paper.

Printed in the United States of America
Bloomington, IN

1stBooks - rev. 06/11/03

ACKNOWLEDGEMENTS

I am grateful for everyone's support in making this book possible. First I'd like to thank Mary Newnam for her editorial review. I am forever grateful to Rev. Eunice Chalfant, Celebration of Life Church for presenting the class on the "Power of Now". The monthly support of my Books and Company Writer's Group was invaluable. They kept me focused on the project. I am also grateful for the support of my friends, and family throughout this process.

*Dedicated to
everyone who has a problem or
has ever had a problem eating consciously*

Contents

Preface ix

Part I: Conscious Levels I-IV 1

    Chapter One 2
    Conscious Eating

    Chapter Two 6
    Conscious Eating— Level I: Planning
    Conscious Eating – Level II: Eliminating Nonfoods

    Chapter Three 9
    Conscious Eating – Level III: Focusing

    Chapter Four 12
    Conscious Eating— Level IV: Observing

Part II: Action 17

    Chapter Five... 18
    Navigating Challenges

    Chapter Six 22
    30 Day Eating Consciously Journal

Part III: Rewards 85

    Chapter Seven... 86
    Sugar Free Desserts

    Chapter Eight 102
    Before and After Story

Appendix 1: Food Plan **108**

Appendix 2: Resources **111**

Appendix 3: Sugar Free Items **112**

Preface

I have 27 years of experience with yo-yo dieting. I lost 90 pounds in two years and maintained the weight loss for nine years. I didn't understand why I had lost it or what it took to maintain the weight loss. In 2002 I lost an additional 20 pounds. The ideas for this book came after I lost the last 20 pounds.

I woke up to what was working after I started living in the present moment. I truly became aware of what I was doing. I understood why I was able to keep the weight off. I understood what I was doing differently than what I had done in the past. And that understanding is what I hope to pass on to you.

Part I: Conscious Levels I-IV

Chapter One

Conscious Eating

We don't want to think about what we're eating. We just want to eat. But if you've been eating excess foods, the only way to change the habit is to first become conscious of exactly what you are eating.

Conscious eating has four levels. The first level is *planning* what you are going to eat. The second level is *eliminating* nonfoods that cause fuzzy thinking, forgetfulness and excessive consumption. The third consciousness level is *focusing* on the food as you consume it. And the final level of consciousness and most powerful is *observing* your own behavior.

This book will take you through the four consciousness levels. It will teach you how to apply each level to your life and provide you with affirmations for each level.

Affirmations are important, because you're teaching yourself to do something different from what you've done in the past. And what really works in maintaining a weight loss is repetition. Repeat, repeat, and repeat! You're repeating your new eating habits. You are changing your life style. You are not going to revert to the way you used to eat.

Influenced by the mass hypnosis, I used to think that if I lost the weight, I could then eat everything I had missed while I was dieting. That's the yo-yo, (the insane) thinking. *If you eat what you always ate, you get what you always got—fat.*

Do You Eat Unconsciously?

I define unconscious eating as eating without being totally aware of what or how much you have eaten. In Webster's New World Dictionary it is defined as not aware of; not realized or intended (an unconscious habit). To find out whether you eat unconsciously, complete the following questionnaire.

Eating Consciously for Natural Weight Loss

Am I Eating Unconsciously?

1. Do you eat even if you are not hungry? Yes ☐ No ☐
2. Do you eat while you are driving your car? Yes ☐ No ☐
3. Do you eat while standing or walking? Yes ☐ No ☐
4. Do you eat so quickly that you feel unsatisfied when you've finished? Yes ☐ No ☐
5. Do you eat while watching television? Yes ☐ No ☐
6. Do you forget what you've eating by the end of the day? Yes ☐ No ☐
7. Do you eat just because someone offered it to you? Yes ☐ No ☐
8. Do you frequently have symptoms of gas or heartburn? Yes ☐ No ☐
9. Have you tried to lose weight before and failed? Yes ☐ No ☐
10. Do you crave specific foods? Yes ☐ No ☐
11. Have you ever eaten an entire cake or pie in one or two days? Yes ☐ No ☐

If you answered yes to one or more questions, keep reading. You may be an unconscious eater.

Why would you want to become a "conscious eater?" Being a conscious eater does not mean "going on a diet." Diets are what people go on and go off. Conscious eating is not a temporary solution. It is a permanent change.

There are at least three distinct benefits of being conscious of what you eat.

1. "Dieting" will be unnecessary.
2. Your body will reduce to its natural size.
3. Your life will be less stressful.

Dieting Will Be Unnecessary

If you think about and are consciously aware of everything you put in your mouth, you will eat less— effortlessly. You won't have to count calories, obsess about the fat grams or weight and measure ad infinitum.

When you start being consciously aware of what you are eating, you may find that some of the foods you thought you liked won't taste the same. Slowing down makes you pay attention to what is going in your mouth. You will become sensitive to quality as well as quantity.

Your Body Will Reduce To Its Natural Size

When you stop obsessing about "dieting" and start being consciously aware of what you are eating, you will achieve what you want! Your body will reduce in size. It won't be like a speeding bullet, but it will happen in time. What's the hurry? When I lost 90 of my 110 pounds of excess weight, it was slow. If I had weighed myself every day, I would have become discouraged and quit being aware. Weigh once a month and don't worry about it. Use the scale as an honesty tool instead of a reason to quit. If the scales don't say what you want it to, ask yourself, "What am I eating that I can change to achieve the results I want?"

Your Life Will Be Less Stressful

If you are more conscious about your food, amazingly you will be more conscious about everything. You will tend to stop trying to do everything at the same time, which will reduce the stress in your life.

To become more consciously aware, you must be willing to:

> Be completely responsible for everything you eat.
> Be different.
> Stay consciously aware when you eat.

You are responsible for everything that goes into your mouth. Don't blame other people or situations. If you say to yourself, "I had to work late, so I stopped by a fast food restaurant, you are still responsible for your action."

I dated a guy once who was a gourmet cook. Everything he cooked was absolutely delicious; melt in your mouth good. But it was loaded with heavy sauces, butter and fat. When I took the responsibility for the quality of what I ate, I had to do the cooking. Sure I could have asked him to change what he was cooking, but it's my responsibility to assure that I eat what's appropriate for me. Me, no one else has that power.

You will be different. You may be called a picky eater. You will have to say no to foods that don't agree with your food plan. Most of us want to be like everyone else. We want to eat everything in sight and still weigh 120 pounds. In my old perception of people, I thought they could eat a ton of food and stay thin. But then I started really observing the thin people around me.

I had a thin friend who often talked about food. She gave elaborate dinner parties and was frequently in the middle of food discussions. I wanted to be just like her, eat all the food I wanted and still be thin. One day I invited her to dinner at my house. When she filled her plate, she picked up the smallest piece of fish, one French fry and two tablespoons of cole slaw. That was my thin, "big eating" friend. In reality, she didn't eat a lot; she talked a lot about food. I've never met a thin person who can eat as much as I did. But, at the time, I didn't know it.

Some people make an effort to be conscious of what they are eating for a few days, and then revert to unconscious eating. To lose weight consistently, you must stick with being conscious. After your new behavior is established, your choices will be different. If you eat a meal unconsciously, stop and ask yourself "what did I just eat?" If you can't remember because you ate it too quickly, *don't* go back for seconds. Slow down. Enjoy and savor each bite.

ABC News did a poll on whether people would eat one-third fewer calories in order to live longer. Nearly three-quarters of Americans in the ABC News polls said that eating fewer calories isn't worth it. [1] Only 25% of Americans are willing to eat less to live a longer and healthy life. It's your choice.

---

[1] Abcnews.go.com/onair/dailynews/agingpoll-020830.html – 9/02/02

Chapter Two

Conscious Eating— Level I: Planning

This level of consciousness requires that you eat only three meals a day with nothing in between, unless your doctor or nutritionist requires you to eat more meals. If you are required to eat more, then eat nothing between those meals. Level I consciousness also requires that you write down what you plan to eat for at least 30 days.

This is the first stage of conscious eating. Be aware of what you are putting in your body. No longer ask yourself "Why am I gaining weight— I hardly eat anything." If you are honest with yourself you will know what you are eating. You won't need to count calories. You will know whether what you are eating will lead to weight gain or weight loss.

How

1. Eat three meals a day unless your doctor or nutritionist requires more.
2. Write down what you plan to eat at least one day in advance for 30 days. Do not change what you eat at this first stage. Become more aware of what you are eating. You may be surprised. Later on, I will provide you with a plan of eating that worked for me.
3. Repeat the following affirmation 30 times silently each morning and 30 times each evening. In addition, write down the affirmation at least 21 times each day. If you experience resistance while you are writing, write your thoughts about the affirmation on the reverse side of your paper. Write everything that comes to mind. When you have run out of resistance thoughts, begin rewriting the affirmation. Follow these same instructions with the affirmations you are given for each consciousness level.

Affirmation

I eat nothing in between meals and I weight ___(insert goal weight) pounds.

Conscious Eating – Level II: Eliminating Nonfoods

Now you're ready for Conscious Eating— Level II. This level may do more for you than anything else you can do. Most people know and accept that refined sugar is not a food group and that eliminating it will not result in a deficiency in any nutrients.

William Dufty wrote a classic on the ill effects of sugar in his book "Sugar Blues." In his book he states:

> "Man-refined sugar is eight times as concentrated as flour, and eight times as unnatural—perhaps eight times as dangerous. It is the unnaturalness that deceives the tongue and appetite, leading to over consumption. Who would eat 2 ½ pounds of sugar beets a day? Yet the equivalent in refined sugar is a mere 5 ounces. Overconsumption produces diabetes, obesity, and coronary thrombosis among other things."[2]

The evidence is available, sugar not only increases cravings, it also has numerous side effects that we'd all like to avoid.

Eliminating sugar from your food plan will give you more energy. While eating sweet, squishy things, you have less room for the more healthy foods, vegetables, or fruits. Apple pie a la mode, hot fudge sundaes, pecan pie a la mode, malted milk balls and chocolate covered peanuts may taste good but the sad thing about all those desserts is you never get as much as you want! One bite isn't enough and a hundred may leave you wanting more, more, and more.

When you kick the sugar habit; the sugar cravings will stop. It may seem weird to eat from necessity and not from what would "be good." A friend of mind calls sugar cravings—food schizophrenia. One voice says, "eat some vegetables", the other voice says "you deserve a special sweet treat today." The sweet treat voice wins more

---

[2] William Dufty, *Sugar Blues* (New York: Warner Books Inc., 1975) P. 216.

often than the quiet vegetable voice until you consciously control it. Taking the sugar out of the equation shuts down your fat twin voice—the voice that is out to kill you with sugar.

An unexpected event may happen when you give up the sugar. Your thinking will become less foggy. For the first time, your thinking will be crystal clear. While consuming massive amounts of refined sugar, you may have thought you were operating at maximum efficiency. After all, you have a good job, and all the accoutrements of a successful person. Nothing is wrong with your mind. You just have a little weight problem.

Give up refined sugar and the roller coaster will stop. The highs and lows will even out. You will become mellower, less irritable. The "Sugar Blues" will be over. You will reach a new level of consciousness. You will know exactly what effects food has on you because you will remember what you've eaten during the day. When you don't feel comfortable after eating, you can identify the culprit. That is conscience eating. Without sugar in your diet, you will be totally aware of what goes in your mouth. Give up sugar and you move to the second level of consciousness. Your thinking becomes clearer, you lessen the chances of chronic illness, you enter an entire new way of living. Take the plunge—eliminate the sugar.

How

1. Read labels on the food you purchase. Eat only foods with sugar listed 5th or lower on the list of ingredients.
2. Eliminate alcoholic beverages such as beer, wine and liquor.

Affirmation

Everything I eat is sugar free or sugar is listed as 5th or lower on the ingredient list.
I weight ___ (insert goal weight) pounds.

Chapter Three

Conscious Eating – Level III: Focusing

Level III of conscious eating involves living in the now. "Living in the now" means becoming consciously aware of the present moment. According to Eckhart Tolle, author of the book, "The Power of Now", you can practice this by taking any routine activity that normally is only a means to an end and giving it your fullest attention, so that it becomes an end in itself. He gives the example of walking up and down the stairs in your house or place of work, paying close attention to every step, every movement, even your breathing.

He goes on to give an example of washing your hands and paying attention to all the sense perceptions associated with the activity: the sound and feel of the water, the movement of your hands, the scent of the soap.[3]

We are always in the present moment. The present moment exists even without our awareness. What we become aware of we can control. If we continually ignore the present moment by thinking about what happened in the past or projecting into the future, we miss the opportunity to live fully in the present moment. Try these exercises for practicing being in the now.

Exercise I

The next time you are driving alone in your car, turn off the radio. Just be totally aware of your hands on the steering wheel, your feet on the accelerator, the speed limit, how fast you are going, the other cars, the scenery, the sounds of the air conditioner or heater, the sounds from outside the car. Notice what you smell. Take in everything from your five senses. Be totally present with the experience of driving.

---

[3] Eckhart Tolle, Practicing The Power of Now (Novato: New World Library) 21-22.

Exercise II

Go for a walk alone in your neighborhood or in a park. Notice the weather. Is it hot, cold, windy, or humid? Look around you. Notice the birds chirping, the insects scurrying around, and other walkers. Notice the smells in your neighborhood; notice the houses, the businesses. Try to be aware of your surroundings. Stay relaxed.

How did you feel after doing these exercises? Write down your feelings. Were you feeling anxious, bored, scared, or lonely? Just be aware of what you felt. The first time you turn off the radio in your car, you may feel a deep hollow feeling, an emptiness that you want to fill with noise. It may even be a little bit scary not to have any sound to distract you.

Eating in the Now

Now that you have practiced staying in the present moment during various aspects of your life, let us move to being present when you eat your meals. What does it mean to be in the now while eating? It means focusing on nothing else but what you are eating. It means turning off all outside stimulants—no television and no radio. It means no multitasking—talking on the telephone and eating at the same time. Your only assignment is to sit down at your table and eat your meal. Just slowly eat your meal without thinking about what happened in the past or projecting what is going to happen in the future. No need to start thinking about your next meal. All you want to do is to eat, enjoy and savor the meal in front of you. Can you do that just for one meal? Try it. You will be totally amazed that you may get bored with eating before you finish your meal. You may actually get full and find that the food is satisfying you nutritionally and filling your need for energy.

How

Pick at least one meal a day that you can eat with no distractions from the television, radio and telephone. Sit down at your table, desk or wherever you eat and eat your meal slowly, consciously and in the present moment.

Affirmation

I eat my meals in the present moment and I weight ___ (insert goal weight) pounds.

Chapter Four

Conscious Eating— Level IV: Observing

This tool not only can affect your food consumption but it can change your entire life. This life-changing tool of consciousness takes you to the level of becoming the observer. It frees you from your unconscious, compulsive mind and gives you the tools you need to really control your life instead of just reacting to it.

Start listening to the voice in your head—the voice that tells you to eat more food; the voice that says "I will start my diet tomorrow." The one that says one small piece of cake or pie won't hurt. Listen. Listen to that voice. The key word is to listen, not **act**. Just observe. Do not tell yourself "I shouldn't be having these thoughts." Do not run from them. Just listen and absolutely avoid judging.

You will find your inner voice to be like that of a child wanting attention. If you pay attention to it and not ignore it, it seems satisfied and dissolves. Remember what you are always told about listening to other people and not trying to solve their problems. That's what your inner voice wants you to do. Just listen. Don't try to solve the problem by putting food in your mouth to shut the voice up. Eating may appear to solve the inner voice's problem, but it will cause you a problem. You ate something you hadn't planned to eat. Now you feel guilty and you ask yourself why not keep eating since you've again blown your resolve not to overeat. And the cycle continues. More food, more weight, more guilt, more remorse. Now the voice is beating you up because you ate.

But you can stop the insanity by just listening, just observing. After all what's the worse thing that could happen to you? There is no way you will die of starvation between lunch and dinner or between dinner and breakfast.

Exercise
The next time you are eating something that you really like-- something that you usually eat to excess, try just listening to the voice that tells you to take another bite even though you know you have had

enough. Try this when you are alone. Not while you are eating with someone else. You don't want any outside distractions. Not other people, not the television, not the radio or a book. This really has to be done alone so you can clearly hear the voice; so you're not eating to please someone else and you can stop when you realize you have had enough. In fact it may be even better to preplan when you are going to stop, in case your body fails to communicate that it is full. Decide in advance how much you are going to eat. Determine what a reasonable portion is and use that amount as your gauge of when to stop. Stop and just listen to the voice. Be very gentle with the voice, but do not move your hands to put more food in your mouth. Remember the only way the food can get in your mouth is if you put it there and you have the power to sit still and just listen. If you just listen this time, you will be totally amazed that the next time you eat the same food, you will stop at a reasonable amount without difficulty. Try it.

How

Plan your meal at least one day in advance. Follow your plan. Listen for the inner voice and just observe what you hear and do not act on any urging to eat something not planned.

Affirmation

I have complete control over what I eat. I weight ___(insert goal weight) pounds.

Eating Consciously 30 Day Plan

The following summarizes and gives you a 30 day plan for incorporating all four levels of consciousness into your life.

Week 1
Level I Consciousness: Planning

Eat at least three meals a day. Eat more if required by your doctor or nutritionist. Write down what you plan to eat at least one day in advance.

Week 2
Level II Consciousness: Eliminating Nonfoods

Continue Level I. Plus only eat foods with sugars listed 5th or lower on the list of ingredients. Eliminate alcoholic beverages such as beer, wine and liquor. Devise meal plans based on sound nutrition. Be aware of your serving size. If you're unsure of how many ounces of protein you need a day or the amount of fruits and vegetables you should incorporate into your meals, please consult a good nutritionist or your doctor.

Week 3
Level III Consciousness: Focusing

Continue Levels I and II. In addition, eat at least one meal a day with no distractions from the television, radio or telephone. Sit at your dining table, desk or wherever you can eat your meal slowly, consciously and in the present moment.

Week 4 +
Level IV Consciousness: Observing

Continue Levels I, II and III. Listen for your inner voice and just observe what you hear. Do not act on any urging to eat something not planned. Immediately forgive yourself if you do. Eat as planned at the next meal.

You may discontinue writing down your meals when it becomes routine. Adjust your food plan, based on an honest assessment of whether it is nutritious, and whether you are losing weight. Only weigh yourself once a month. Do not worry if the weight comes off slowly. You are changing your life style, not dieting.

So many people ask me specifically what I ate to lose weight. The food plan I received from my Overeater's Anonymous-How sponsor is in Appendix 1. Consult your doctor or nutritionist before you follow this or any other food plan. This one worked for me because it eliminated refined sugar and reduced the amount of simple carbohydrates I consumed. Remember it is a plan, not a straight jacket. Decide on your bottom line. Just because a food is not listed doesn't mean that you can't eat it. You may want your bottom line to be no refined sugar with at least 3 meals a day. Allow yourself to eat anything else without guilt and judgment. Remember you must be able to forgive yourself if you do not follow your plan exactly. Forgiveness allows you to follow your plan at the next meal, instead of waiting for the next time you want to go on a "diet." The only thing that is required is total awareness and honesty with yourself about what you eat. No one else is judging you but you. If you do get judgments from other people, it's none of your business.

Louistine Tuck

Part II: Action

Chapter Five

Navigating Challenges

As with everything, there will be challenges along the way to conscious eating. Situations will occur in your life that will make you want to give up eating consciously. But there is a solution—Level IV Consciousness. This level of consciousness can overcome any obstacles to conscious eating.

Hunger Pangs

The first hunger pangs may occur when you come off the sugar. It may be a hunger pang or a craving. Sometimes it's difficult to distinguish which is which. When you have a hunger pang and it's not even close to the time you are scheduled to eat, what should you do? The usual response to that question is to distract yourself with something else—drink some water, chew gum. In the early stages of going off sugar, I suggest you do just that, but after you've followed the 30 day plan for a while and you get hungry in between meals, you should ask yourself a simple question. Why am I hungry? When you ask yourself that question, you will learn what's really bothering you, and it has nothing to do with food. Use the hunger pang as an opportunity for self-discovery.

Allow the hunger pang to be a signal to learn what's really bothering you, not as a signal to eat. Hunger pang? What am I feeling? Why am I hungry? What am I really hungry for— food or comfort?

More

What do you do when you want more to eat than what is on your plate— when you want to go back for seconds, thirds? This is a perfect opportunity to use Level IV consciousness. You planned ahead what you were going to have for a meal, but your inner voice is telling you that it wasn't satisfying, that you need more. What do you do? You listen to your inner voice. You don't judge it and say you shouldn't feel this way or have those kinds of thoughts. Just observe the thoughts, but do not act on them. You will be amazed that the thought will just dissolve. It may be difficult the first time, but hang in there, do not give up. The desire for more will dissipate.

Pushers

Who are pushers? Pushers are your friends, family and loved ones who offer you food in between meals, sugary baked goods and second helpings. They love you, and they are not trying to sabotage your food plans. But it's up to you to respond to their efforts with a firm no thank you. It's not their job to keep you on your food plan. It's yours. You teach people how to treat you.

Do not say, "I'm on a diet." You're not on a diet. You've changed your lifestyle. Diet says temporary to people, so they're just waiting for you to go off your diet. But if you never use the word diet, never think the word diet, you never set up the expectation for going off it.

Emotions

One of the things that happen when you stop stuffing yourself with food is that all sorts of emotions flow. When you eat unconsciously, you may only feel two emotions, sad when you are not eating and happy when you are. Now you will feel everything.

Emotions are scary when you have unwittingly suppressed them with food. We also live in a society that tells us not to feel. My idol when I was growing up was Jackie Kennedy because she didn't cry at her husband's funeral. I thought that was just the coolest thing, so controlled. But now I know that emotions are not to be suppressed but released.

If our emotions don't show on our faces, we end up wearing our emotions as excess food. We pay a steep price for our stoicism. Emotions are meant to flow in and out of our bodies. But if we stuff them down with excess food, they get stuck there and we're depressed and unhappy without a clue to the cause.

So what is one to do with emotions? Use the forth level of consciousness to observe the emotion, becoming a silent witness to the emotion. Do not act on the emotion; just allow the emotion to be without judgment. Emotions dissolve, exiting the body, for unconscious eaters, usually through the stomach. That's why we get confused and think we're hungry all of the time, when the real problem is an emotion trying to escape our bodies.

Exercise

Do this exercise when you are alone or with a trusted friend. Sit in a comfortable chair. Allow yourself to think of something in your past or present that gives you great pain—the death of a loved one, the loss of a relationship, a divorce. Think about what you have avoided thinking. One thing at a time. Allow the feeling to come up. Instead of just crying about it, observe yourself thinking about it. Use the Fourth level of consciousness to become the observer of you having the emotional reaction to a painful incident in your life. Keep breathing. Allow the emotion to bubble up. Notice as you observe the painful thoughts, they begin to dissipate. Do not divert yourself from thinking about it. Allow yourself to feel the emotion and observe how you feel as the silent witness, the observer. Observe yourself being yourself. The pain will dissolve into nothingness. It cannot hurt you; it is only a series of thoughts.

Witnessing feelings can be difficult. But if you don't deal with your feelings, they will just keep replaying. Eradicate old buried emotions by finally experiencing them in the now.

Other Unconscious Behaviors

If you are unconscious about food, when you become a conscious eater, sometimes other unconscious behaviors surface. You may find that you are a compulsive shopper, spender or debtor. At first you may not recognize it, after all you need all those clothes to go with your thinner body. But if you keep buying, long after you have a closet full of the new sized clothes or you're buying things you don't even need, your unconsciousness may have slipped into the money arena.

You may start being unconscious with your computer. Staying on the computer for hours and hours. Playing games repeatedly. Surfing the web until you're seasick. The mind that refuses to stay present finds all sorts of escapes from reality. But the escape route can be closed with Level IV consciousness. Whatever unconscious behavior you are experiencing can end with conscious attention. Silently witness the behavior, decide how much is enough and stop. Witness how you feel when you stop. Just observe your feelings but do not take any action to continue and the compulsion to play one more game, buy one more suit, will dissolve.

This sounds so simple and it works. Try it and your life will gradually change. You will be able to face whatever life presents you with one moment at a time.

Chapter Six

30 Day Eating Consciously Journal

    This journal will help you get through the first 30 days of Eating Consciously. It takes a month to lock in a habit. So, for the next 30 days, stop and look at what you're focusing on in your life, outside of losing weight and say "not now" to as many things as you can. Were you going out of town for a purpose other than business? Postpone it. Do you regularly meet your friends for lunch? Wait until you have your new habits in place. Treat the changes you're making to reach your weight loss goals as the most important thing in your life for the next 30 days.

    Follow the instructions given for each day. On the 31st day, please call or e-mail me and let me know how you are doing. I want to know if this plan works for you.

Louistine Tuck
louistinetuck@sbcglobal.net
(937) 436-5769

Affirmation

I eat nothing in between meals and I weigh ___pounds.

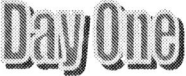

The infinite is in the finite of every instant.
Zen Saying

Instructions
Level I Consciousness: Planning

1. Eat at least three meals a day. Eat more if required by your doctor or nutritionist.
2. Write down what you plan to eat at least one day in advance. Do not change what you eat the first 7 days. Become more aware of what you are eating.
3. Write the affirmation—*I eat nothing in between meals and I weigh ___(insert goal weight) pounds* —21 times on the opposite page.

MENU PLAN

Breakfast

Lunch

Dinner

Affirmation

I eat nothing in between meals and I weigh ___ pounds.

Day Two

The best part of our lives we pass in counting on what is to come.
William Hazlitt

Instructions: Repeat Day One instructions.

MENU PLAN

Breakfast

Lunch

Dinner

Affirmation

I eat nothing in between meals and I weigh ___pounds.

Day Three

We are always getting ready to live, but never living.
Ralph Waldo Emerson

Instructions: Repeat Day One instructions.

MENU PLAN

Breakfast

Lunch

Dinner

Affirmation

I eat nothing in between meals and I weigh ___ pounds.

Day Four

The future is purchased by the present.
Samuel Johnson

Instructions: Repeat Day One instructions.

MENU PLAN

Breakfast

Lunch

Dinner

Affirmation

I eat nothing in between meals and I weigh ___ pounds.

Louistine Tuck

Day Five

***The best thing you can do for the future is to live
with everything you have in the present—Ralph Marston Jr.***

Instructions: Repeat Day One instructions.

MENU PLAN

Breakfast

Lunch

Dinner

Affirmation

I eat nothing in between meals and I weigh ___pounds.

Day Six

I do not think "tomorrow" or "later" or "another time." I think now.
-For Today-

Instructions: Repeat Day One instructions.

MENU PLAN

Breakfast

Lunch

Dinner

Affirmation

I eat nothing in between meals and I weigh ___ pounds.

Louistine Tuck

Day Seven

*What is actual is actual only for one time
And only for one place. —T.S. Eliot*

Instructions: Repeat Day One instructions.

MENU PLAN

Breakfast

Lunch

Dinner

Eating Consciously for Natural Weight Loss

Affirmation

Everything I eat is sugar free or sugar is listed as 5th or lower on the ingredient list. I weigh ___ pounds.

Day Eight

Every situation—nay, every moment—is of infinite worth; for it is the representative of a whole eternity. —Johann Wolfgang von Goethe

Level II Consciousness: Eliminating Nonfoods

1. Continue Level I Consciousness: Planning
2. Read labels on the food you purchase. Eat only foods with sugar listed 5th or lower on the list of ingredients. Devise a meal plan based on sound nutrition. Review the food plan I've provided in Appendix I and consult a nutritionist or your doctor to determine if it is safe for you to use.
3. Write down the following affirmation—*Everything I eat is sugar free or sugar is listed as 5th or lower on the ingredient list. I weigh ___(insert goal weight) pounds*—21 times on the opposite page.

MENU PLAN

Breakfast

Lunch

Dinner

Affirmation

Everything I eat is sugar free or sugar is listed as 5th or lower on the ingredient list. I weigh ___ pounds.

Day Nine

Above all, we cannot afford not to live in the present.
Henry David Thoreau

Instructions: Repeat Day Eight instructions.

MENU PLAN

Breakfast

Lunch

Dinner

Affirmation

Everything I eat is sugar free or sugar is listed as 5th or lower on the ingredient list. I weigh ___ pounds.

Louistine Tuck

Day Ten

To take what there is, and use it, without waiting forever in vain for the preconceived—to dig deep into the actual and get something out of that—this doubtless is the right way to live. —Henry James

Instructions: Repeat Day Eight instructions.

MENU PLAN

Breakfast

Lunch

Dinner

Affirmation

Everything I eat is sugar free or sugar is listed as 5th or lower on the ingredient list. I weigh ___ pounds.

Day Eleven

Let him who would enjoy a good future waste none of his present
Roger Babson

Instructions: Repeat Day Eight instructions.

MENU PLAN

Breakfast

Lunch

Dinner

Eating Consciously for Natural Weight Loss

Affirmation

Everything I eat is sugar free or sugar is listed as 5th or lower on the ingredient list. I weigh ___ pounds.

Louistine Tuck

Day Twelve

Tomorrow's life is too late. Live today.
Martial

Instructions: Repeat Day Eight instructions.

MENU PLAN

Breakfast

Lunch

Dinner

Affirmation

Everything I eat is sugar free or sugar is listed as 5th or lower on the ingredient list. I weigh ___ pounds.

Day Thirteen

With the Past as past. I have nothing to do: nor with the Future as future I live now and will verify all past history in my own moments.
Ralph Waldo Emerson

Instructions: Repeat Day Eight instructions.

MENU PLAN

Breakfast

Lunch

Dinner

Affirmation

Everything I eat is sugar free or sugar is listed as 5th or lower on the ingredient list. I weigh ___ pounds.

Day Fourteen

The more you are able to honor and accept the NOW,
The more you are free of pain and suffering.
Eckhart Tolle

Instructions: Repeat Day Eight instructions.

MENU PLAN

Breakfast

Lunch

Dinner

Affirmation

I eat my meals in the present moment and I weigh ___ pounds.

Day Fifteen

Face Everything And Recover (FEAR)
Unknown

Level III Consciousness: Focusing

1. Continue Levels I and II.
2. Eat at least one meal a day with no distraction from the television, radio or telephone. Sit down at your table, desk or wherever you eat and eat your meal slowly, consciously and in the present moment.
3. Write down the following affirmation—*I eat my meals in the present moment and I weigh ___ (insert goal weigh) pounds*—21 times on the opposite page.

MENU PLAN

Breakfast

Lunch

Dinner

Affirmation

I eat my meals in the present moment and I weigh ___ pounds.

Day Sixteen

Do not dwell in the past, do not dream of the future, concentrate the mind on the present moment.
Buddha

Instructions: Repeat Day Fifteen instructions.

MENU PLAN

Breakfast

Lunch

Dinner

Affirmation

I eat my meals in the present moment and I weigh ___ pounds.

Day Seventeen

He is blessed over all mortals who loses no moment of the passing life in remembering the past.
Henry David Thoreau

Instructions: Repeat Day Fifteen instructions.

MENU PLAN

Breakfast

Lunch

Dinner

Affirmation

I eat my meals in the present moment and I weigh ___ pounds.

Day Eighteen

When you are not aware in the present moment, you have no power.
Gary Zukav and Linda Francis

Instructions: Repeat Day Fifteen instructions.

MENU PLAN

Breakfast

Lunch

Dinner

Affirmation

I eat my meals in the present moment and I weigh ___ pounds.

Louistine Tuck

Day Nineteen

The butterfly counts not months but moments, and has time enough
Rabindranath Tagore

Instructions: Repeat Day Fifteen instructions.

MENU PLAN

Breakfast

Lunch

Dinner

Affirmation

I eat my meals in the present moment and I weigh ___ pounds.

Day Twenty

There are no problems only situations to be dealt with now, or to be left alone and accepted. –Eckhart Tolle.

Instructions: Repeat Day Fifteen instructions.

MENU PLAN

Breakfast

Lunch

Dinner

Affirmation

I eat my meals in the present moment and I weigh ___ pounds.

Day Twenty-One

If we live primarily in the past, we waste the present and preempt the future. –Michael A. Williams

Instructions: Repeat Day Fifteen instructions.

MENU PLAN

Breakfast

Lunch

Dinner

Affirmation

I have complete control over what I eat. I weigh ___ pounds.

Day Twenty-Two

Yesterday is history. Tomorrow is a mystery.
Today is a gift. That's why it's called the present.
Unknown

Instructions
Level IV Consciousness: Observing

1. Continue Levels I, II and III.
2. Listen for the inner voice and just observe what you hear and do not act on any urging to eat something not planned. Forgive yourself if you do. Eat as planned at the next meal.
3. Write down the following affirmation—*I have complete control over what I eat. I weigh ___(insert goal weight) pounds*—21 times on the opposite page.

MENU PLAN

Breakfast

Lunch

Dinner

Affirmation

I have complete control over what I eat. I weigh ___ pounds.

Day Twenty-Three

Live and savor every moment, this is not a dress rehearsal.
Unknown

Instructions: Repeat Day Twenty-Two instructions.

MENU PLAN

Breakfast

Lunch

Dinner

Affirmation

I have complete control over what I eat. I weigh ___ pounds.

Louistine Tuck

Day Twenty-Four

***The only form of life that hangs onto the past is man.
Raymond Charles Barker***

Instructions: Repeat Day Twenty-Two instructions.

MENU PLAN

Breakfast

Lunch

Dinner

Eating Consciously for Natural Weight Loss

Affirmation

I have complete control over what I eat. I weigh ___ pounds.

Day Twenty-Five

*When you live in complete acceptance of what is,
that is the end of all drama in your life.*
Eckhart Tolle

Instructions: Repeat Day Twenty-Two instructions.

MENU PLAN

Breakfast

Lunch

Dinner

Affirmation

I have complete control over what I eat. I weigh ___ pounds.

Louistine Tuck

Day Twenty-Six

The master gives himself up to whatever the moment brings.
Lao Tse

Instructions: Repeat Day Twenty-Two instructions.

MENU PLAN

Breakfast

Lunch

Dinner

Eating Consciously for Natural Weight Loss

Affirmation

I have complete control over what I eat. I weigh ___ pounds.

Louistine Tuck

Day Twenty-Seven

I freely let go of the past. I freely let go of that which yet will be.
I am a now person in a now experience.
Raymond Charles Barker

Instructions: Repeat Day Twenty-Two instructions.

MENU PLAN

Breakfast

Lunch

Dinner

Affirmation

I have complete control over what I eat. I weigh ___ pounds.

Louistine Tuck

Day Twenty-Eight

The moment is timeless.
Ram Dass

Instructions: Repeat Day Twenty-Two instructions.

MENU PLAN

Breakfast

Lunch

Dinner

Affirmation

I have complete control over what I eat. I weigh ___ pounds.

Day Twenty-Nine

No matter what time it is, it is always now.
Marianne Williamson

Instructions: Repeat Day Twenty Two instructions.

MENU PLAN

Breakfast

Lunch

Dinner

Eating Consciously for Natural Weight Loss

Affirmation

I have complete control over what I eat. I weigh ___ pounds.

Day Thirty

When you accept what is, every moment—that is enlightenment.
Eckhart Tolle

Instructions: Repeat Day Twenty-Two instructions.

MENU PLAN

Breakfast

Lunch

Dinner

Affirmation

I am grateful for increasing health, and vitality.

Day Thirty

Our deepest fear is not that we are inadequate.
Our deepest fear is that we are powerful beyond measure.
Marianne Williamson

Instructions:

Continue writing down your meals until it becomes routine. Adjust your food plan based on an honest assessment of whether it is nutritious and you are losing weigh. Only weigh yourself once a month. Remember this is a lifestyle change.

Menu Plan

Breakfast

Lunch

Dinner

Part III: Rewards

Chapter Seven

Sugar Free Desserts

Giving up refined sugar does not mean that you will never have dessert again. It means your desserts will contain natural or artificial sweeteners. After you have been off sugar for a few months natural sweeteners will taste heavenly. I recommend you wait until you have been free of refined sugars at least a month before you try these recipes. Enjoy.

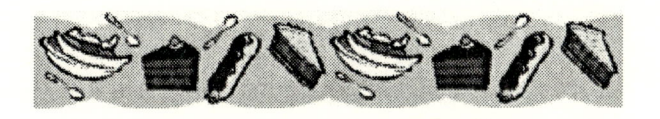

Apple Raisin Pie

4 medium apples, peeled and sliced
¼ cup raisins
2 tablespoons all fruit apricot jelly
¼ cup flour
¼ teaspoon salt
⅛ cup pineapple juice
1 teaspoon cinnamon
1 pie crust unbaked

Preheat oven to 350 degrees

1. Combine all ingredients and place into pie dish.
2. Put on top crust. Make 4 slits on the top of the crust
3. Bake at 350 degrees for 50 minutes.

Servings: 8

Louistine Tuck

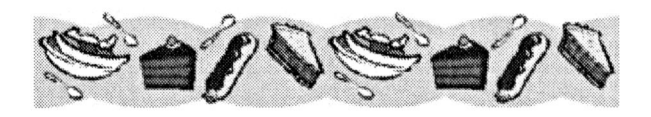

Banana-Apple Smoothie

1 ½ cup soy milk
1 frozen banana, sliced
4 cubes frozen apple juice
1 teaspoon coconut flavor
5 dates, sliced

1. Freeze apple juice in an ice cube tray.
2. Slice and freeze 1 banana.
3. Combine all ingredients in a blender. Blend until smooth.

Servings: 1

Eating Consciously for Natural Weight Loss

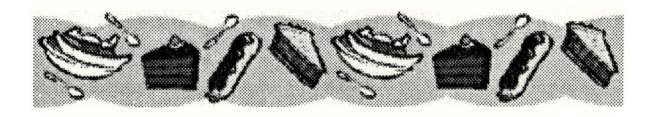

Banana-Date Bread

1 packet of yeast
½ cup warm water
2 mashed bananas
2 cups whole-wheat flour
1 teaspoon vanilla
½ teaspoon salt
½ cup soy butter
2 tablespoons all juice apricot jelly
1 cup pitted dates, chopped
1 cup walnuts, chopped
½ cup pineapple juice

Preheat oven to 350 degrees

1. Stir warm water, and yeast together in a small bowl.
2. Set aside in a warm place for 10 minutes.
3. Mash the bananas in a mixing bowl.
4. Stir together the remaining ingredients including the warm water and yeast in the bowl.
5. Pour into a greased 9x5 bread pan, and bake at 350 degrees for one hour

Servings: 8

Adapted from recipe in Country Life Vegetarian Cookbook, p. 63

Louistine Tuck

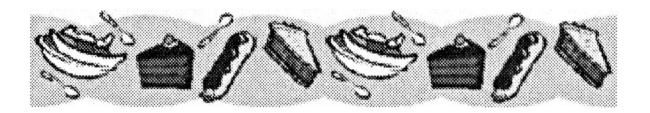

Carob Brownies

1 cup carob powder
1 cup whole wheat or spelt flour
1 cup walnuts
¼ cup oil
2 teaspoons vanilla
4 tablespoons all fruit apricot jelly
½ teaspoon salt
½ cup applesauce

Preheat oven to 350 degrees

1. Mix all ingredients together in a bowl.
2. Oil an 8" x 8 pan and pour ingredients into pan.
3. Bake at 350 degrees for 30 minutes.

Servings: 9

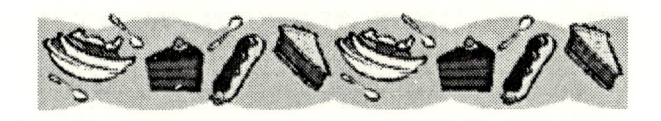

Carob Chip Cookies

2 cups oatmeal
1 cup applesauce
2 teaspoons vanilla extract
¼ cup vegetable oil
1 cup raisins
½ cup walnuts, chopped
½ cup non-dairy carob chips

Preheat oven to 375 degrees.

Mix all the ingredients together in a large bowl.
Spoon batter onto a lightly oiled cookie sheet, forming 24 cookies.
Bake 12-15 minutes at 375 degrees.
Allow cookies to cool before removing from the cookie sheet.

Servings: 24

Adapted from recipe in Simply Vegan, pp.109-110

Louistine Tuck

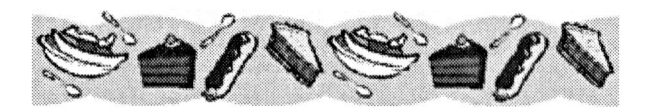

Carrot Cake

1 cup pineapple juice
¼ cup vegetable oil
½ cup water
1 packet dry yeast
2 tablespoons honey
2 cups whole-wheat flour
½ teaspoon salt
1 teaspoon cinnamon
¼ teaspoon nutmeg
1 teaspoon vanilla
1 cup raisins
½ cup chopped walnuts
1 ½ cups carrots

Preheat oven to 375 degrees.

Stir together pineapple juice and oil. Set aside.
Stir warm water, dry yeast and honey together in a small bowl. Set aside in warm place for 10 minutes.
Stir together flour, salt, cinnamon, and nutmeg, vanilla, raisins, walnuts and carrots.
Gently stir wet ingredients into dry ingredients.
Pour into an oiled 8 x 8 pan, and bake at 375 degrees for 15 minutes. Reduce heat to 350 degrees for 40 more minutes. Serve cooled with Cream Cheese Frosting.

Servings: 8

Cream Cheese Frosting

1 cup soy cream cheese
1- ½ tablespoons margarine
2 tablespoons all fruit apricot jelly
2 teaspoons vanilla

1. Place all ingredients in food processor or blender.
2. Blend until smooth and spread on carrot cake.

Adapted from recipe by Jeanine DuBois

Louistine Tuck

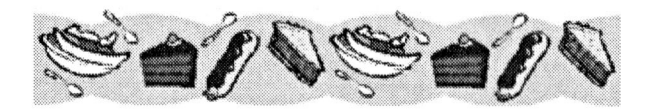

The Elvis Cookie

3 ripe bananas
2 ½ cups oatmeal
1 ¼ cup raisins
1 cup walnuts (optional)
¼ cup vegetable oil
4 ½ tablespoons peanut butter
1 ½ teaspoon vanilla
½ teaspoon salt

Preheat oven to 350 degrees

Mash two bananas in a mixing bowl.
Add remaining ingredients.
Stir until all ingredients are combined.
Let mixture rest for 10 minutes.
Measure out 2.5 ounces of mixture and place in a bar pan or shape into bars in a regular cookie sheet pan.
Cook for 25 minutes or until the bars are golden brown on the bottom.

Servings: 14 bars

Adapted from recipe in Country Life Vegetarian Cookbook, p. 50.

Eating Consciously for Natural Weight Loss

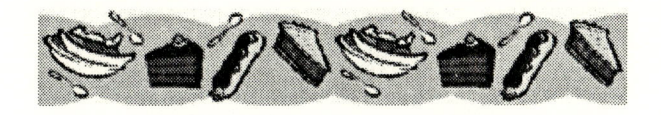

Mango Smoothie

1 frozen banana, sliced
1 cup pineapple juice
1 mango, peeled and sliced

1. Slice and freeze 1 banana
2. Combine all ingredients in a blender.
3. Blend until smooth.

Servings: 1

Louistine Tuck

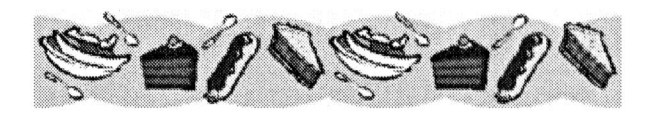

Oatmeal- Raisin Cookies

1 cup applesauce
1 cup raisins
2 cups rolled oats
½ cup walnuts (optional)
¼ cup oil
1 teaspoon vanilla
½ teaspoon salt

Preheat oven 350 degrees

1. Combine and mix all ingredients in a bowl.
2. Let mixture sit for 10 minutes. Drop into lightly oiled cookie sheet by spoonfuls.
3. Bake for 25-30 minutes or until bottoms are golden brown.

Servings: 20

Eating Consciously for Natural Weight Loss

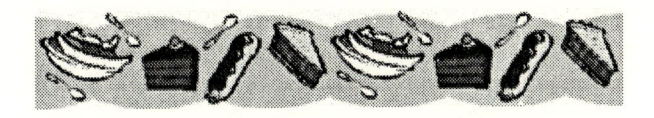

Pineapple Ice Cream

1 cup pineapple juice
2 tablespoons non-dairy milk powder
1 frozen banana
4 ice cubes

1. Place all ingredients in a blender.
2. Blend until smooth. Serve soft or freeze

Servings: 1

Adapted from recipe in Vegetarian Tasting 2002, p.69

Louistine Tuck

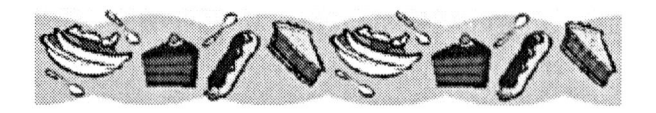

Pumpkin Pie

1 can (16 ounces) pumpkin
1 teaspoon cinnamon
½ teaspoon salt
½ teaspoon ground ginger
⅛ teaspoon ground cloves
¼ cup vegetable oil
2 tablespoons all fruit jelly
⅛ cup pineapple juice
1 pre-made piecrust

Preheat oven to 400 degrees

1. Place all ingredients in a food processor. Blend until smooth.
2. Pour into pre-made piecrust pan.
3. Bake for 30 minutes at 400 degrees. Reduce to 350 and bake 30 more minutes, until the center of the pie is firm. Allow the pie to cool for 30 minutes, then refrigerate for 1 hour.

Servings: 8

Eating Consciously for Natural Weight Loss

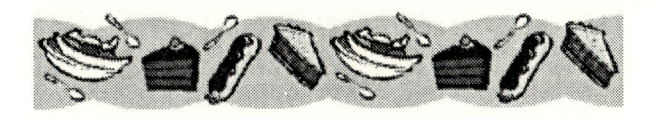

Sweet Potato Bars

2 ripe bananas
2 cups mashed sweet potatoes
2 cups oatmeal
1 cup raisins
½ cup walnuts (optional)
¼ cup vegetable oil
2 teaspoons cinnamon
1 teaspoon vanilla
1 teaspoon nutmeg
½ teaspoon salt

Preheat oven to 350 degrees

1. Mash two bananas in a mixing bowl.
2. Add remaining ingredients.
3. Stir until all ingredients are combined.
4. Let mixture rest for 10 minutes.
5. Measure out 2.5 ounces of mixture and place in a bar pan or shape into bars in a regular cookie sheet pan.
6. Cook for 25 minutes or until the bars are golden brown on the bottom.

Servings: 14 bars

Adapted from recipe in Country Life Vegetarian Cookbook, p. 50

Louistine Tuck

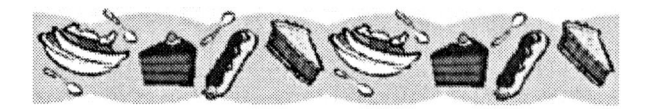

Sweet Potato Pie

3 medium-large potatoes (microwave or boil)
2 bananas
1-teaspoon cinnamon
1-teaspoon nutmeg
1 tablespoon vanilla flavor
¼ cup vegetable oil
2 tablespoons all fruit apricot jelly
⅛-cup pineapple juice
1 pre-made piecrust

Preheat oven to 400 degrees.

1. Place sweet potatoes and bananas in a food processor. Blend until smooth.
2. Add remaining ingredients to food processor and blend.
3. Pour into the pre-made piecrust pan.
4. Bake for 30 minutes at 400 degrees. Reduce to 350 and bake 30 more minutes, until the center of the pie is firm. Allow the pie to cool for 30 minutes, then refrigerate for 1 hour.

Servings: 8

Adapted from recipe In the Kitchen with Rosie, pp 112-113

Eating Consciously for Natural Weight Loss

Before Pictures

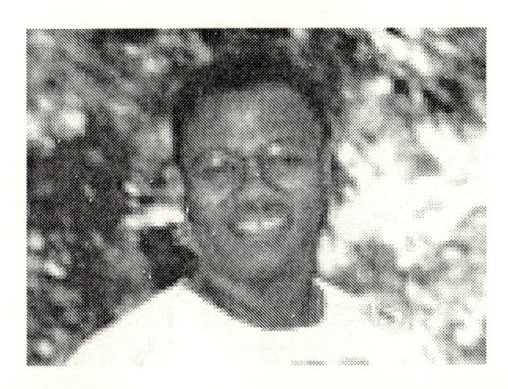

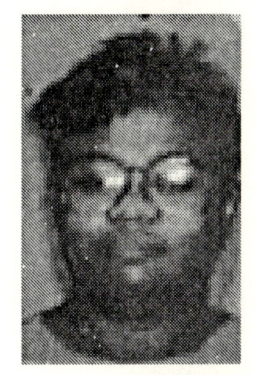

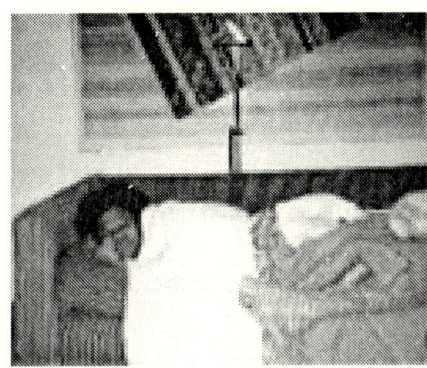

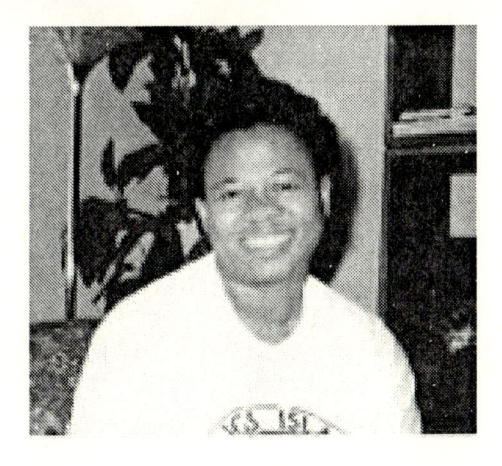

Chapter Eight

Before and After Story

Over a 2-year period, I lost 90-95 pounds and managed to keep it off for nine years. But I was scared all of the time. I thought just one extra bite and all of the weight would come back on. I became a support group junkie. I went to support meetings six out of seven days a week. I was compulsive about everything. As soon as one compulsive behavior was removed, another would crop up. Sometimes I'd hit two to three meetings a day. Fear kept me going back. Sometimes I would forget which meeting I was in and identify myself as belonging to another group. So around and around I went.

On January 2002, I got off the merry-go-round. It happened in a most unexpected way. I signed up for the Power of Now class given at my church. I was a little reluctant to sign up, because I thought I already knew all there was to know about being in the "Now." After all, one of the premises of the support groups I attended was "live one day at a time." But I pushed my hesitation aside and decided to attend the class. The first week of the class I got a terrible cold and couldn't go, but I purchased "Practicing The Power of Now" by Eckhart Tolle. Every word resonated with me. I morphed the book, took notes, bought Tolle's companion book "Practicing the Power of Now."

To say my life changed is an understatement. From the time I was a very young person, I had a problem with compulsive behaviors, overeating, shopping till I dropped, dating without ceasing. Always looking for something or someone to assuage my need for spiritual fulfillment. Tolle said, "As you listen to your thoughts, you feel a conscious presence—your deeper self—behind or underneath the thought. The thought then loses its power over you and quickly subsides... This is the beginning of the end of involuntary and compulsive thinking."[4] After reading that passage in the book, I knew that just maybe I could do something about stopping all of my

---

[4] Eckhart Tolle, Practicing The Power of Now (Novato: New World Library) 19.

Eating Consciously for Natural Weight Loss

compulsive behaviors. I started practicing living in the **now**, the present moment as often as possible.

Each week at the class I had a new "**now**" discovery. One week I discovered that by being very present with the food I was eating, that it expanded and filled my stomach much quicker than ever before. I no longer felt compelled to eat one extra bite. I started practicing eating in the **now** with most of my meals and lost 20 additional pounds. I also discovered that if my ego had other ideas about what I was going to eat, that if I just observed the thoughts without taking any actions, the thoughts would leave.

During a guided visualization at one of our Sunday services, I visualized sharing what I had learned. So I started working on putting together a workshop on Conscious Eating in the **Now**.

Developing the workshop required skills I didn't know I had. In the past, I would have stopped at the idea stage and just wailed, "I don't know what to do," and let the idea drop. But this time, I sat in front of my computer, stayed in the **now**, and everything I needed to know came to me either as an inspirational thought, a hunch, intuitively or through friends. I have now given five workshops, and I have four more scheduled through 2003.

My "before" isn't rosy. As early as the ninth grade, I started trying to lose weight. I only weighted about 125 pounds, but I still was teased at school and at home. My stepfather called me chubby; the boys at school nicknamed me oink-oink. I believed them and set out to do something about it. I attempted the workout route, lost a few pounds and stopped working out.

In the 11th grade, I tried Dr. Atkins' protein diet and lost about 20 pounds so quickly I still thought I was fat. The only way I knew I had lost weight was through my clothes. I remember buying size 3's. I have a picture of me at the prom and I looked downright anorexic before it was a recognized eating disorder. But of course I got all sorts of compliments about the weight I had lost.

By the time I was in college, all the weight was back on. I don't know what it is about late night cramming, but it always screams for greasy fried chicken. As a reward for all my studying, I yielded to the cry for fried greasy foods.

I don't remember my exact weight when I graduated from college but it was enough to make me think I had to do something to get it off. After graduation, I moved to Washington, D.C., lived in a rooming house on Dupont Circle and proceeded to attempt to lose the pounds I had gained at college. A friend of mine, in D.C. working and living at the same rooming house fasted on the weekends for religious purposes. I started fasting with her to lose weight. It was also a convenient way to save money since meals weren't served between lunch on Saturday and breakfast on Monday mornings. Weekend starvation worked. I lost the excess pounds. But of course I was in the yo-yo diet syndrome and my weight crept back up over the next year.

The next thing I tried in 1974 was Weight Watchers. I thought I was a humongous size, but my top weight was 150 pounds. I lost all my so-called excess weight—30 pounds and weighed 120 pounds for five minutes. I immediately began to regain the weight as soon as I received my lifetime membership pin. I stopped going to the meetings and started the cycle all over again.

I tried Weight Watchers again, using an alias. I had this thought that the same diet never worked twice. Perhaps a new name would trick my mind and I could lose the 16 pounds I had gained in about 6 months. Didn't work. Next on my list of diets was eating only things with fructose in it. That lasted a minute. I think I lost 10 pounds.

Then I tried hypnosis. Friends at work had been reporting all of their good results through hypnosis. So I gave it a try too. The hypnotist sat me down in a homey looking room and programmed my mind to believe that starchy foods tasted like paste and sugary foods were disgusting. I could immediately feel the difference. Just thinking about some of my favorite binge foods made me want to gag. I had a few follow-up sessions with the hypnotist, but to my disappointment instead of him hypnotizing me, he put in a tape of his voice. After about four sessions, he gave me a tape of him and told me to play it when I needed a booster. The hypnotism lasted about a year and after that I deliberately made myself eat some of the offensive food and the spell was broken.

After coming out of the hypnotism spell, I didn't try to diet for a while. Oh, yes I did. I now remember that I read a book about eating anything you want, no matter what. After eating everything and anything you wanted, the next stage was to quit punishing yourself for wanting so much of it and you would automatically start eating reasonable amounts and lose weight. Didn't work for me. I started

Eating Consciously for Natural Weight Loss

eating giant chocolate chip cookies every day. They were the size of a dinner plate. This wasn't all I ate. I still ate all my usual meals, plus a couple of giant cookies. I never lost my taste for them and I didn't lose any weight either.

After I became pregnant with my daughter, I stopped all diets. For the first time, I really ate everything I wanted. I was pregnant right? I deserve to treat myself r-e-a-l special. And of course I was eating for two, or was that three people. I gained more weight than I had ever gained before. I was totally out of control. In the past I could control myself enough to stop eating when the scales hit 150 pounds, but not this time. I kept gaining until I weighted 200 pounds. I thought I'd lose the weight after my baby came. Not so. I gained even more. I remember people kept asking me months after I'd given birth, if I'd had my baby.

A friend had heard about a support group for overeaters (Overeaters Anonymous) and she didn't just tell me about it, she took me to meetings. I remember going to the meetings for about a month. Every meeting I went to, I cried. I didn't know why I was crying and I hated crying. I was brought up with the belief that only wimps cried and I didn't like acting wimpy with tears. Even though I started losing weight immediately, I got scared and quit going to the meetings, because the weight came off too easily. Plus, I couldn't stop crying.

My next excursion into the weight loss game was with behavior modification. It worked on changing basic behavior like writing down my food, drawing pictures of my body image, eating slowly and taking at least 20 minutes to eat a meal so that my stomach would get the message that it was full. I lost about 20 pounds on this program. I was down to about 180. We had a celebration dinner at the end of the class to practice our new skills. I remember wishing that my fellow classmates weren't with me so I could really eat what I wanted instead of sticking with the programmatically correct selections.

I kept the 20 pounds off, but I wasn't satisfied. The weight seemed to have hit a plateau. The answer came through Oprah. In the late eighties, Oprah lost a lot of weight with the Optifast Program and I wanted to duplicate her results. However Optifast was an expensive diet program and I really couldn't afford it. If I paid for the program, I would have to make a lot of financial sacrifices in other areas of my life, so I decided to pray about whether I should bite the bullet and do

Optifast. When I prayed, I heard a still, small voice say O. A. I asked "O.A.?" "I don't want to do O. A., I want to do Optifast." I thought God had gotten the message mixed up. Despite God's mix up, I decided to give O.A. a call. I was really hesitant because my policy was to never repeat diet programs. I especially didn't want to repeat a program that touched me emotionally.

The closest meeting to me was a HOW O.A. meeting. So I trudged to my first HOW meeting. I immediately knew I was in the right place. I asked a lady to sponsor me and she agreed. I did 30 days of questions and stayed abstinent from sugar and white flour. The weight started dropping off. But this time, I didn't run from O.A., because I wasn't crying. The group was huge; I sat in the back of the room, didn't open my mouth and just did what everybody else was doing. I kept at it for a year and lost about 40 pounds. Did I keep it off? No. Did I keep going to meetings? No. I wasn't through learning.

I not only didn't keep the weight off, I gained almost triple the amount I had lost. After four years, of eating to my stomach's discontent, I weighed 230 pounds. But the weight didn't take me back to O. A. I didn't go back until I got the connection between food and my mental attitude. I finally understood that my behavior, emotions and mental clarity were affected by what I consumed. So I returned to O. A., not just to lose weight, but to regain my sanity.

And regain my sanity, I did. I lost 90 pounds of the weight I had gained over the four years. It was a slow process. But I remained consistent in my eating plan. I ate 3 meals a day with nothing in between and no refined sugar. I attended two to three O. A. meetings a week, I sponsored other people and I did service for the organization.

I was convinced that I would always be a compulsive overeater. One of the things the A.A. Big Book says is that we will never grow new legs. So I thought that meant I would never recover from my compulsion. My deeper healing began—with the power of living in the now. For this one moment, I am no longer a compulsive person. And a moment is all I have in the eternally present now.

Eating Consciously for Natural Weight Loss

After Pictures

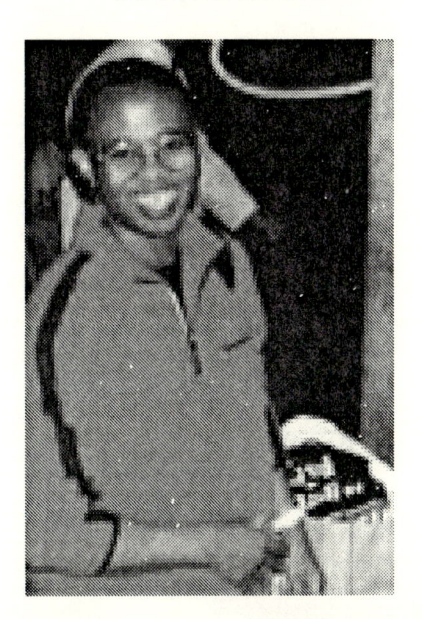

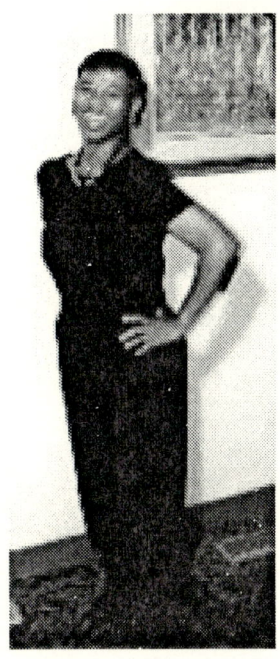

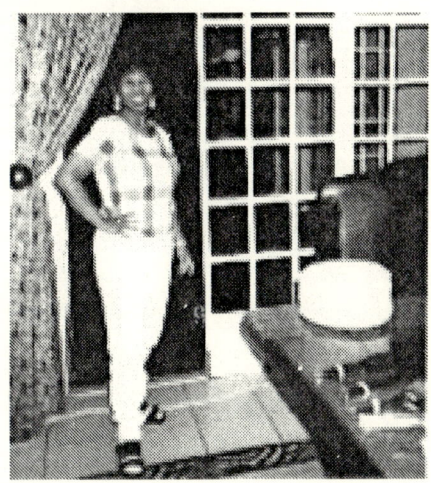

Appendix 1: Food Plan[*]

Breakfast	Lunch	Dinner
1 protein 1 fruit choice 1 carbohydrate 1 teaspoon fat (optional)	1 protein 2 vegetable choices 2 tablespoons salad dressing (optional) 1 teaspoon fat (optional)	1 protein 3 vegetable choices 2 tablespoons salad dressing (optional) 1 teaspoon fat (optional

Food Choices

Protein Group	Vegetables	Vegetables
Beef – 4 oz Chicken – 4 oz Pork – 4 oz Lamb – 4 oz Fish – 4 oz Turkey – 4 oz Veal – 4 oz Liver – 4 oz Eggs – 2 Hard cheese – 2 oz Curd or cottage Cheese – 1 cup Tofu – 12 oz 2 % Milk, Buttermilk, Yogurt – 2 cups	<u>1 cup</u> Alfalfa Sprouts Artichokes Asparagus Bean Sprouts Bok Choy Broccoli Brussels Sprouts Cabbage Cauliflower Celery Chard Cumbers Eggplant Greens Lettuce Mushrooms Okra	Oriental Vegetables Peppers Radishes Parsley Parsnips Pickles (unsweetened) Sauerkraut String Beans Summer Squash (yellow, Crookneck, spaghetti) Tomatoes Turnips Water Chestnuts Zucchini

---

[*] This food plan is not endorsed or sanctioned by Overeaters Anonymous. Before using this or any other plan consult your doctor or nutritionist.

Eating Consciously for Natural Weight Loss

Half-cup	Vegetables	
Beets Carrot	Onions Pumpkins	Yellow turnips Winter Squash

Fruits	Fruits	Condiments
Apricots – 3 medium Apples – 1 Blackberries – ½ cup Blueberries – ½ cup Boysenberries – 1 cup Fruits (cont.) Cantaloupe melon – ½ Cranberries – 1 cup Gooseberries – 1 cup Grapefruit – ½ Lemons/Limes – 2	Nectarines – 1 Oranges – 1 Pineapples 1 cup or ¼ Fresh Peaches – 1 Fruits (cont.) Plums - 2 Raspberries – ½ cup Rhubarb – 1 cup Strawberries – 1 cup Tangerines – 2	All spices; onion soup; salsa; tamari, soy and Worcestershire sauce; pizza, taco, tomato and Spaghetti sauce Fats Butter, margarine, oil, mayonnaise, salad dressing

Carbohydrate Choices 2 slices whole grain bread 2 cups popped popcorn 1 oz cereal 1 medium potato	Each equals 1 carbohydrate ½ cup brown rice ¼ cup corn meal 1 cup cooked oat meal ½ cup peas	½ cup flour ½ cup corn ½ cup legumes

Vegetarian Food Plan

Breakfast	Lunch	Dinner
1 fruit selection 1 dairy/vegetarian protein	1 dairy/vegetarian protein 2 vegetable selections 2 tablespoons salad dressing (optional) 1 teaspoon fat (optional)	1 dairy/vegetarian protein 2 vegetable selections 2 tablespoons salad dressing (optional) 1 teaspoon fat (optional)

Dairy Protein 2 oz hard cheese 1 cup cottage cheese 2 cups yogurt 2 cups 2% milk 2 eggs Vegetarian Protein 1 whole grain + 1 legume 1 whole grain + ½ dairy protein 1 legume + ½ dairy protein 12 oz tofu 2 tablespoons peanut butter Whole Grains ½ bagel 1 biscuit ½ cornbread + beans	1-2 slices bread ½ English muffin 1 roll ½ cup stuffing ½ cup macaroni ½ cup noodles ½ cup spaghetti 1 oz dry cereal ½ cup cooked cereal ½ cup rice + beans 2 cups plain popcorn 1 tortilla Legumes ½ cup beans ½ cup black eyed peas 1 tablespoon peanut butter ½ cup lentils 6 oz tofu

Appendix 2: Resources

Reading List

Sugar Blues – William Dufty
Suffering is Optional – Cheri Huber
The Power of Now – Eckhart Tolle
Practicing The Power of Now – Eckhart Tolle
The Heart of the Soul – Gary Zukav and Linda Francis

Power of Now Groups

Celebration of Life Church
4100 Benfield Drive
Kettering, OH 45429
1st Monday of the Month
Noon

Support Groups

Overeaters Anonymous
Overeatersanonymous.org

Life Coach

Louistine Tuck
Hownow Seminars
(937) 436-5769
louistinetuck@sbcglobal.net

Appendix 3: Sugar Free Items or Sugar Listed as 5th Ingredient

Salad Dressings

Creamy Ranch (Kroger)
Lite Creamy Ranch (Kroger)
Classic Caesar (Kraft)
Seven Seas Italian Dressing (Kraft)
Mamma DiSalvo's Authentic Salad Dressing
Newman's Own Family Recipe Italian
Newman's Own Ranch Dressing
Marzetti Garden Ranch Dressing
Wishbone Asian Sesame
Wishbone Oriental
Blue Cheese (Any Brand)

Jelly/Preserves

Smucker's Simply 100% Fruit
Kroger's Just Fruit
Polaner All Fruit

Ketchup

Estee Ketchup

About the Author

Louistine Tuck writes this book from experience. For over 27 years she yoyo dieted. She'd lose weight, keep it off for a few months and regain all the weight, plus more. She has maintained a 90 pound weight loss for nine years. She lives in Dayton, Ohio with her daughter and conducts workshops and seminars on Eating Consciously for Natural Weight Loss.

Printed in the United States
1232900005B/238-300